HOW TO
UNPLUG
YOUR CHILD

101 Ways to Help Kids Turn Off Their Gadgets and Enjoy Real Life

LIAT HUGHES JOSHI

HOW TO UNPLUG YOUR CHILD

This edition copyright © Liat Hughes Joshi, 2025
First published in 2015

All rights reserved.

No part of this book may be reproduced by any means, nor transmitted, nor translated into a machine language, without the written permission of the publishers.

Liat Hughes Joshi has asserted their right to be identified as the author of this work in accordance with sections 77 and 78 of the Copyright, Designs and Patents Act 1988.

Condition of Sale
This book is sold subject to the condition that it shall not, by way of trade or otherwise, be lent, resold, hired out or otherwise circulated in any form of binding or cover other than that in which it is published and without a similar condition including this condition being imposed on the subsequent purchaser.

An Hachette UK Company
www.hachette.co.uk

Vie Books, an imprint of Summersdale Publishers
Part of Octopus Publishing Group Limited
Carmelite House
50 Victoria Embankment
LONDON
EC4Y 0DZ
UK

www.summersdale.com

This FSC® label means that materials used for the product have been responsibly sourced

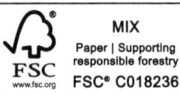

The authorized representative in the EEA is Hachette Ireland, 8 Castlecourt Centre, Dublin 15, D15 XTP3, Ireland (email: info@hbgi.ie)

Printed and bound in Poland

ISBN: 978-1-83799-481-6

Substantial discounts on bulk quantities of Summersdale books are available to corporations, professional associations and other organizations. For details contact general enquiries: telephone: +44 (0) 1243 771107 or email: enquiries@summersdale.com.

Disclaimer
Neither the author nor the publisher can be held responsible for any loss or claim arising out of the use, or misuse, of the suggestions made herein. Parental supervision is recommended for all the activities in this book.

CONTENTS

Introduction
4

Food and Cooking
89

Indoor Fun
10

Science and Nature
100

Get Outdoors
42

Activities on the Go
110

Arty and Crafty
68

A Few More Ideas...
119

INTRODUCTION

---

*Screens are part of life
but shouldn't become life itself.*

Technology is thoroughly ingrained in all our lives and our children's lives are no exception. From an early age, screens are a key source of entertainment for them and, like it or not, highly effective at keeping them occupied. By the school years, they're needed for homework and are being used ever more in the classroom – no longer just for IT/computing lessons. Once our offspring reach the teenage stage, their social worlds would surely stop spinning without social media and messaging on whichever app is the hip thing of the moment.

But sometimes it can all get too much. Sometimes wouldn't you appreciate a little downtime from the technological torrent that eats into our offline relationships? To actually talk to each other and do things together that don't involve texting and messaging, tapping and swiping? If this is how you feel, this book

Introduction

might just help to unglue their eyes from those screens a shade more often.

No one is suggesting turning those gadgets and TVs off altogether or banning them – this would likely be impossible anyway as we need them for so many everyday activities – but it's certainly wise to keep a lid on their use.

How much IS too much then?

Other than for the youngest children, recommending a set daily time limit isn't especially helpful when there is such diversity in what they're actually doing on their screens nowadays. Kids' online time can be recreational, educational, social and functional and there's a huge contrast between watching a wildlife documentary or researching your homework and playing a frankly mindlessly violent game, plus plenty in the middle of these extremes.

It's surely more sensible to discern between good and bad screen activities and then limit these specifically. Define what they can do by category and roughly for how long daily – so, for example, "You're allowed to use the games console and/or apps for an hour and can have 30 minutes of TV." Keep an eye on things; look out for signs of overload and let them know that if they push it or start getting too obsessed and addicted, you can and will reduce their access.

Babies and toddlers

The early years are a crucial time for emotional and verbal development, so it's especially unwise to take any chances in the baby and toddler years. Although the American Academy of Paediatrics recommends no screen time at all for this age group, realistically toddlers find some TV and apps entertaining and there are moments in life when we parents need screens to give us a short break so we can get on with things. It's wise, though, to limit babies and toddlers to no more than an hour a day and keep that hour to decent quality programmes, designed specifically for this age group.

Try not to let handing over a smartphone or tablet become your default "keep them occupied" activity every time you're in a café or on a long car journey – no TV programme or app can be a substitute for talking to your baby or toddler.

And for teenagers?

At the other end of the age scale, this phase deserves special mention, too, as the challenges of getting them away from screens magnify considerably, partly because they have their own gadgets, their social lives rely on messaging and it can be difficult to police their time online when they're not with you. Plus, as well as using gadgets for longer spells, teenagers have a tendency to frequently nip onto their phone to message a friend or fleetingly check Instagram or TikTok.

Set ground rules about sensible usage, e.g. not after a certain time at night, during homework unless directly relevant and not at the dinner table.

On top of that, watch for warning signs that screens are causing problems – limiting social skills in person or impacting their sleep – and cut back accordingly if they are.

And of course this book has ideas for offline activities with teen appeal, some so good they might even want to post about them afterwards…

How to use this book

This is all about reminding the kids that you don't have to be stuck to screens to have fun, but equally you probably have neither the time nor the inclination to turn yourself into some sort of jolly, home version of a children's party entertainer. Nor do you want to be spending a fortune buying special kit.

All of the activities in this book are free or require fairly minimal equipment beyond what would normally be found in a typical family home. Some of the ideas do need parental input but how much will depend on your kid's age and skill levels.

A few of them involve some internet or gadget usage beforehand as a kick-starter – realistically that is the quickest way to get instructions – but the heart of all of these activities is very much offline.

Some activities will be one-offs – after they've done it once, your child probably won't want a repeat run – but we hope others will become firm favourites.

Introduction

Some handy things to keep at home

If you're really going to get stuck into this book, there are a few activities requiring common kit that's worth stocking up on or keeping the next time some comes your way:

- Craft scissors
- Large cardboard boxes
- Strong glue
- Coloured paper and card
- Blank greetings cards

INDOOR FUN

- COMPUTER
- **IMAGINATION**

Indoor Fun

SIGN LANGUAGE CHALLENGE

DIFFICULTY: ■■■□□

Learning basic sign language is relatively easy, a useful life skill and surprisingly appealing – especially if your child does so with friends and they can then use it to communicate together. Fingerspelling is an undaunting starting point – single signs for individual letters that can be used to spell out words. If they get into this, they could progress on to learning whole word signs.

What you'll need

- A sign language guide (online is fine!)

Semaphore is another, more unusual skill if they enjoy this...

FIND THE MOST EMBARRASSING OLD FAMILY PHOTOS

DIFFICULTY: ●○○○○

Dig out those long-neglected snaps from the attic and challenge your child to find the top three most embarrassing/amusing ones from days of yore. Prepare for much sniggering at your clothes and hairdos and comments of the "but you looked soooo young there, Mum"/"you had hair then, Dad..." variety.

What you'll need

- A pile of old pics or albums

You could stage a mock mini-award ceremony for the most cringeworthy outfit in a photo or worst hairstyle with home-made certificates or mini silver foil-crafted "Oscars".

CHARADES

DIFFICULTY: ▮▮▯▯▯

OK, *you* might have played this hundreds of times during your childhood Christmases, but for your offspring it's probably still pretty fresh and fun. Pick a theme – films/TV is popular – and divide players into two teams. One person acts out words or phrases to their team-mates each round, with a timer providing a limit. Award points for correct guesses or make the winners the team with the lowest total time used for all their turns together.

What you'll need

- An egg timer/phone timer
- At least four people to make up two teams

The old ones are (sometimes) the best – they've stood the test of time for good reason.

BATH TIME AT THE WRONG TIME

DIFFICULTY: ●○○○○

Having a bath at completely the wrong time of day, with no rush to get to bed, keeps small children content for a spell when it's throwing it down outside and they've already watched quite enough TV.

What you'll need

- A bath
- Some waterproof toys and containers

Part of the appeal of this activity is that it's completely free and can be done anytime, but you can add some variety and extra interest by buying some cheap but non-toxic bath goo, crayons or special mouldable foam soap.

DIY SPA DAY

DIFFICULTY: ∎∎▢▢▢

When there's no queue for the family bathroom, let teens set up a "spa" at home. Hair and face masks can be knocked up with typical kitchen ingredients, such as yoghurt, oats, banana, honey, avocado and chocolate. Salt or sugar scrubs are simple to put together too. Enthusiastic experimenters can concoct their own formulations.

What you'll need

- Kitchen ingredients
- Tubs/bowls
- Mixing spoons
- Mask and scrub recipes (these can be found online)

This is perfect for a girly sleepover; let them have some friends over and spend the evening creating and using their spa potions.

CREATE A PERSONAL TIME CAPSULE

DIFFICULTY:

Find a box file and give it to your child to decorate and fill with lists of their dreams and goals for ten years' time. They can also add photos and mementos of their life at the moment. It must then be well sealed and hidden away by a parent ready to be opened in the future – bringing back a flood of memories and insights.

What you'll need

- Pens
- Paper
- A box
- Sticky tape
- Some photos

POWER OFF FOR A NIGHT

DIFFICULTY: ●○○○○

This is a one-off rather than something most of us would do on a regular basis: powering down not just gadgets but the lights and TV, too, can tick boxes for its novelty factor. Allow only wind-up torches and candles (supervised for younger ones), grab a pack of cards or some board games and tell spooky stories. Sweeten the blow of no screens and lights with the promise of a takeaway dinner – after all, the oven will be out of bounds too!

What you'll need

- Candles and torches
- Games that don't require mains electricity

Useful to show children just how reliant we are on electricity for entertainment and daily life.

LEARN A NEW LANGUAGE

DIFFICULTY: ıllll

Challenge yourselves to learn a new language as a family over a set period and see how far you can all get with it. If you're going abroad for a summer holiday, you might want to choose the destination's language. If your child already learns one or two at school, perhaps encourage a more obscure option. Esperanto, anyone?

What you'll need

- A "teach yourself" book and other materials, e.g. CD, for whichever language you've chosen. Online resources can be fantastic for language learning too – definitely an example of the potential positives of screens.

The younger children are when they start to learn another language the better, but remember that some languages are easier than others to pick up.

THEMED PHOTO SHOOT WITH FRIENDS

DIFFICULTY:

A photo shoot where they have to gather props and costumes and make a temporary backdrop on a wall or booth requires plenty of preparation. Theme the shoot around vintage, grunge, silly hats, clashing clothing or a favourite book or film – whatever appeals.

What you'll need

- An old white sheet or large paper roll for the backdrops
- Fabric/marker pens for any scene they want to create
- Masks, specs, interesting tops – raid the charity shop or grandparents' attics for props and costumes

---

A simple alternative: everyone draws a face/shoulders self-portrait on A4 paper then positions it in front of their face for a pic.

SET UP A BOOK CLUB

DIFFICULTY: ■■◌◌◌

This is ideal for some quality parent and child time – if they are old enough to read and you can find books that appeal across generations – or for encouraging older kids to set up a club with a group of like-minded friends. This could focus on an appropriate genre, such as sci-fi or comedy.

What you'll need

- Books!

Don't shy away from e-readers for kids – they bring the added benefits of an integrated dictionary and the ability to download new books instantly. Just watch out for screen glare before bedtime on reading apps on smartphones or tablets – it can hamper sleep, so pick a dedicated e-reader if possible.

INDOOR BALLOON SPORTS

DIFFICULTY: ❙❙◌◌◌

Kids not allowed to play ball games in the house, but it's chucking it down outside? Balloons shouldn't smash the ornaments or windows (although choose the most suitable and spacious room in the house just in case) so allow the kids to let off steam and use them to play sporty activities including volleyball and tennis. A piece of string will do as a net for either. Work on achieving the longest rally or have a match.

What you'll need

- A balloon
- Some string
- Some paper or plastic plates for "tennis rackets"
- Sticky tape
- Lolly sticks

FILM A MUSIC VIDEO

DIFFICULTY: ▋▋▋▋▋

Whether hip hop, pop or even classical floats their boat, putting together a music video can let kids explore their style while they rock on. They can choose outfits, come up with a dance routine, mime to a favourite soundtrack or sing and play instruments if they've got the requisite skills and kit. Alternatively, they could make their own cardboard instruments or simply "air guitar" away to their heart's content!

What you'll need

- Instruments and soundtracks if needed
- Suitable outfits and accessories
- Materials and props to make a set if they want to go that far

---

This activity obviously requires a gadget for filming, but the core of it is sociable, musical and offline.

LEARN THE UKELELE

DIFFICULTY: ▌▌▌▌▌

... or the harmonica, drums or recorder. What we're looking for here is an instrument that anyone can make a half-decent sound from, right from the first blow, strum or bash. You can often buy beginner sets with a "how to play" book, CD or DVD to get going. This is another activity worth allowing screens into as there are lots of fantastic video tutorials online.

What you'll need

- An instrument (check out charity shops for second-hand ones to keep costs down)
- How-to tutorials

Learning an instrument can boost self-esteem, concentration and brain power. Enthusiasts could turn this into a social pursuit by starting a band with friends.

CARDBOARD STAIR SLIDING

DIFFICULTY: ■■□□□

Fend off bad-weather cabin fever with a stair slide. Unfold a large appliance box and lay it along one side of the staircase (those of a nervous disposition can use the bottom steps only rather than the whole length. Those of a very nervous disposition should probably skip this activity altogether…). Stuff cushions/rolled-up blankets onto each step to smooth things under the cardboard so it doesn't buckle. Tape the cardboard to the first step you intend to use (use masking tape as it's less likely to damage anything). Kids could race cars or balls down before sliding themselves.

What you'll need

- At least one very large cardboard box (two will help smooth things out), masking tape and a staircase. Also a very considerable pile of pillows, cushions and duvets to soften landings at the bottom and to stuff under the card.

Indoor Fun

BOARD GAMES NIGHT

DIFFICULTY: ▮▮▯▯▯

Whether they're toddlers or teens, sometimes the thing our offspring crave the most is our attention, and getting down on the floor playing games with them is a huge hit. Put the gadgets down (yes, yours too), place those chores on hold (the washing up can wait) and dust off some board games for the evening.

What you'll need

- Family classics such as *Scrabble*, *Cluedo*, snakes and ladders, dominoes and *Connect4*
- Pizza for half-time
- A score sheet if you're making a tournament out of it

Board games are brilliant for getting family members of different ages together and talking (and, OK, sometimes squabbling, too, but still...).

A GOOD OLD GAME OF CARDS

DIFFICULTY: ■■◦◦◦

A pack of cards still has the power to provide hours of entertainment for Generation Tech and hey, that small deck of 52 is more portable than the lightest tablet. Gin rummy and whist are great for kids, and perhaps poker for teens. Speed – of the card game variety – is especially addictive and appeals to those who might be accustomed to a fast pace of play from all their online gaming.

What you'll need

- A pack of cards
- Knowledge of card games or a book of game rules

Draft the grandparents in for this if they're around and willing – they'll almost certainly recall a few great games from their own childhoods to teach the youngsters.

Indoor Fun

BUILD AN INDOOR FORT

DIFFICULTY: ▍▍▍▍▌

Cluster the furniture in the living room and pile on sheets and quilts to make their very own kingdom.

They'll be scuttling off in there with a torch, books or toys before you know it. And yes, eventually they might end up in there with the tablet but at least the making of it all lured them offline first.

What you'll need

- Some chairs and a table to act as posts
- Sheets and quilts for cover
- Cushions for inside
- A torch, if it'll be dark in there

Making the space strictly kids-only brings a fun exclusivity to this one – it's all about marking out some space as their own.

FIND A PEN PAL

DIFFICULTY: ▮▮▯▯▯

Children love getting post of their own and writing to a pen pal is a stealthy but effective way of working on literacy, communication and potentially foreign language skills. Ask around for a pal with shared interests, or it could be a cousin, a friend's child or a former classmate living overseas.

What you'll need

- A pen pal
- A stationery set (take them to the shops to choose an appealing one)
- Supply of stamps

Even the tech generation can get enjoyment out of sending good old-fashioned letters... it's kind of retro. Another idea is to send a message in a bottle.

START YOUR OWN MAGAZINE

DIFFICULTY: ●●●○○

Budding journalists can set their minds to compiling a magazine. It could be about their hobby or an end of year (academic or calendar) review – what were their highlights and memories? Younger ones who struggle with writing could focus on scrapbooking and using photos or drawing pictures.

What you'll need

- Paper
- Pens
- Printed photos
- A stapler to bind the pages together

Of course, they could write a blog or digital magazine but at least get them to mock it up offline.

DOMINO RUN

DIFFICULTY: ❙❙❙❘❘

Invite friends with their own dominoes over and see how big a run they can create. After they've got the hang of basic runs without knocking them down (top tip: leave strategic gaps and fill these in at the end so only a small part can tumble accidentally), they can make all sorts of features, including spirals, staircases and spelled-out words.

What you'll need

- A LOT of dominoes
- Materials to make obstacles and extras, such as ramps (building bricks would work for this)
- A good deal of patience and concentration

The core of this activity is offline, but pique their interest with some of the amazing domino run videos online before they start. Older kids could record theirs for social media afterwards too.

Indoor Fun

CONSTRUCT A HOUSE OF CARDS

DIFFICULTY: |||||

Another charmingly low-tech activity, building a house of cards can be frustrating but engrossing. Start by making an upside down V with two cards about 5 cm apart at the bottom, make more Vs, about 1 cm apart, and then begin adding your horizontal layer on top for a second storey to sit upon. Just don't let anyone sneeze in the vicinity.

What you'll need

- A pack of decent quality, newish playing cards (creased, bent old ones won't do for this)
- A flat non-slip surface as a base

In 2010 American architect Bryan Berg spent 44 days creating a card house replica of the world's largest casino – The Venetian in Macao – inside the casino itself, using over 218,000 cards with no glue.

PAPER AEROPLANE RACES

DIFFICULTY: ▮▮▯▯▯

There are numerous paper aeroplane folding styles – find a few variations and then hold some races between the same and different designs. Hang a hula hoop or another target up somewhere and see if your child can get their plane through, or hold a plane relay race if you've got a gang of kids about the house.

What you'll need

- Paper
- Colouring pens/crayons for decoration
- A tape measure to assess race winners
- Prizes for the most aerodynamic/furthest travelling plane

Adding a competitive element raises this to a new level and decorating the planes brings some art and design into play.

STAGE A TV-STYLE SINGING COMPETITION

DIFFICULTY: ▮▮▯▯▯

Karaoke competitions are nothing new but give it a twist by holding one in the style of their favourite TV singing contest. They'll need a bubbly presenter complete with "microphone" (any old hairbrush does the job), to build a "stage" with a low stool or steps and, if they've the time and inclination, to make a set. Judges could dress and act as famous names from those Saturday night shows. This is great for a party or sleepover.

What you'll need

- Song sheets or a karaoke machine/app
- Stage area
- Different outfits
- Earplugs for nearby grown-ups!

Singing not their thing? Broaden it into a talent show and they can tell jokes or dance instead.

A FAMILY MURDER MYSTERY

DIFFICULTY: ▮▮▮▯▯

Set up a family whodunnit – make up your own clues and characters or download a pre-made version and collect up the necessary props and outfits. Best kept for older children and teens, who'll understand the rules, the need for non-disclosure by the "murderer" and the storyline.

What you'll need

- A murder mystery story
- Props

Getting participants to dress up and to stay in character during dinner enhances the sense of occasion.

CUSTOMIZE YOUR *MONOPOLY* SET

DIFFICULTY: ▮▮▮▯▯

Cover a *Monopoly* board with paper ready for your new version. Select a theme – your local area, football teams or even cat or dog breeds. These then replace the "official" street names and need grouping into colour-coded sets. Make fresh Community Chest/Chance cards or new counters and replacements for the houses and hotels in keeping with the theme. Stick with the original monetary values, though, as otherwise the game might become too short or long.

What you'll need

- Stationery supplies, including paper, card and pens
- A *Monopoly* set

For more fun: see if they can make custom versions of other favourite board games – there are no limits.

LEARN TO JUGGLE

DIFFICULTY: ıı❙❙❙

Juggling never fails to impress and is not quite as hard to master as it looks. There are usually instructions provided with juggling ball sets or ask a friend or relative with the necessary skills if they're willing to teach your child. After they have mastered the three ball/bag throw, your child might even want to learn tricks and more complicated manoeuvres. Practise away and they'll soon have people enthralled by their circus-style talents... next stop a unicycle?

What you'll need

- Juggling balls or bean bags

Once the juggler in the family is confident with bean bags or balls, see what else they can juggle – within reason. Perhaps not your most precious, fragile ornaments...

RETRO PARTY GAMES FOR TEENS

DIFFICULTY:

Invite some friends round for a retro games party and play all those "they should be too old for" favourites. Pass the parcel, blind man's buff, musical chairs, pin the tail on the donkey (you could change this to pin the nose on the celebrity photo) all take on a different dimension when you're 15 instead of five. They do need to be past the "that's babyish" stage, though.

What you'll need

- Presents with teen appeal for pass the parcel
- Some chairs
- A blindfold for blind man's buff
- A list of games and their rules if it has been too long since they were little to remember them

---

Being given an excuse to find their inner child that, secretly, your teen hasn't wanted to let go of, can be fun.

FOREHEAD DETECTIVE

DIFFICULTY: ▍▍▕▕▕

Stick the name of a famous person, object or animal on each player's forehead, either in turn or all at once. They aren't supposed to see or be told who they "are" and must ask questions of others to identify their persona. Only yes/no answers are permitted and no mirrors are allowed, so watch out for sneaky folk heading to the bathroom to see what's written on their note.

What you'll need

- Post-it/sticky notes
- A pen

You could have pairs of well-known people, so Barack and Michelle Obama, Ant and Dec or William and Kate, and ask players to find their partner as well once they have worked out who they are.

THE "WHAT'S MISSING" GAME

DIFFICULTY: ●○○○○

Collect at least ten random small objects on a tray, ask one player to study the tray, then remove one thing when they aren't looking and ask them to identify what's disappeared. Selecting objects for the tray is as time-consuming as the game itself – encourage them to find several similar but slightly different items to add to the challenge.

What you'll need

- A tray and some objects. Choose a room that's quite busy with belongings – it doesn't work so well in a minimalist space.

An alternative is to do this on a whole room scale – ask a player to leave the room and then move or hide an item.

SOCK PUPPET SHOW

DIFFICULTY: ▮▮▯▯▯

Breathe new life into unloved, unpaired socks with decorations such as buttons, lengths of wool and felt pieces (fabric glue saves on the sewing). Once they're made, let the show begin! The smallest family members will delight in a little sock puppetry and can act out anything that their imagination creates.

What you'll need

- Socks to make the puppets, decorations and fabric glue, and a little set and stage can be fashioned from a large shoebox or old cereal boxes.

Using puppets lets children explore all kinds of characterizations and is amazing for young imaginations.

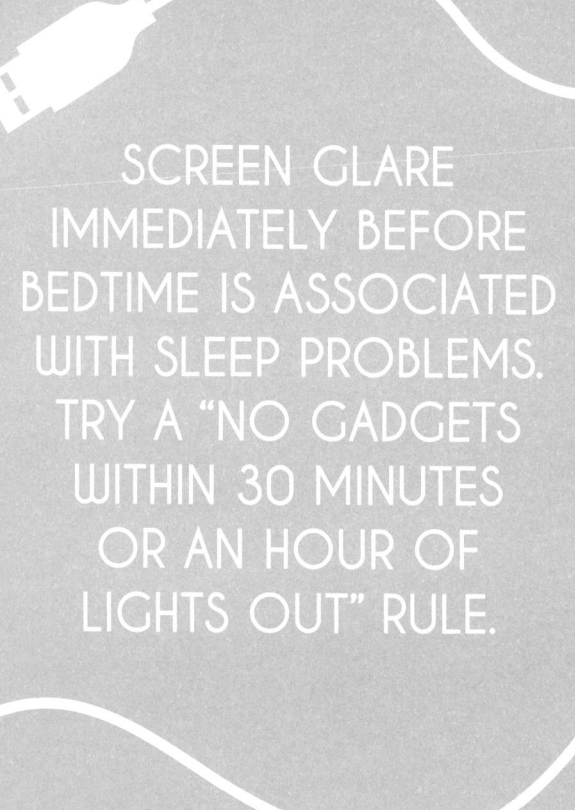

GET
OUTDOORS

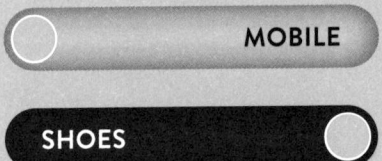

A DOG FOR THE DAY

DIFFICULTY: ◼◼◻◻◻

Assuming you don't have one of your own, borrowing a canine chum can drag animal-loving youngsters away from screens and out for "walkies". Ask friends with pooches, or look at one of the websites that match borrowers with owners needing dog walking/sitting. Ensure children are accompanied by an adult if they're younger, inexperienced with dog care or the pet isn't well known to you.

What you'll need

- A dog that's used to children
- Its lead and poop bags
- Some doggy treats to maximize tail wagging

Dog owners will sometimes offer a fee for walking – something to bear in mind for older offspring who are responsible enough to take a dog out alone and want to earn some extra cash.

GARDEN CAMPING

DIFFICULTY: ▮▮▯▯▯

All the upsides of camping (the fresh air, the novelty!) minus the communal bathrooms and forgetting to take the tent pegs.

An evening toasting marshmallows on a campfire or barbecue and telling stories by torchlight has a fighting chance of getting them to leave those screens inside (hide them and turn your router off if necessary). Given you might all get woken every hour by foxes and at 6 a.m. by the dawn chorus, stick with non-work/school nights for this one.

What you'll need

- A garden, or, if you don't have one, persuade the grandparents or some friends to host
- Typical camping gear – buy second-hand or borrow to keep costs down

ICE MARBLES

DIFFICULTY: ●●○○○

These look beautiful sitting amid snow but you do need some very cold weather to hit. When it does, fill balloons with water and add some bright food colouring, tie the top of each one and put them outside on a sub-zero night. By morning they'll freeze – snip off the balloon plastic and the result: colourful ice marbles.

What you'll need

- Sub-zero temperatures
- Balloons
- Water
- Food colouring

If it's not quite cold enough to rely on ice forming outside, cheat by using your freezer if there's space. The kids can then keep an eye on how long the finished product takes to melt outside through the day.

SAND SCULPTING

DIFFICULTY: ▊▊▊▊▊

Who says you have to stick with building castles at the beach? The trick to making sand sculptures – be they of animals, letters, cars – is to mix in a lot of water with the sand, creating a muddy consistency. Start off with more basic creations and work up. Look online for ideas before you leave and even older cynics will be heading for the beach before you can say "don't forget the sunscreen".

What you'll need

- A trip to the beach (or a sandpit for smaller creations at home)
- Buckets (for water as well as sand)
- A selection of other containers of varying sizes – cups, tubs, etc.
- Tools, e.g. spade, knives, spoons, spatula

Something for older offspring who need a new twist on sandcastle building.

WATER-TASTIC GAMES

DIFFICULTY: ●○○○○

Grab some water pistols, soak a few kitchen sponges in a bucket, make water balloons, turn that garden sprinkler on (provided there isn't a hosepipe ban at the time), then chuck the kids outside in their swimwear on a hot day and await the soggy mayhem.

What you'll need

- Some water pistols, balloons, sponges, hosepipe and sprinkler
- Definitely a few towels for afterwards!

For more fun, try a game of water balloon catch: see how many times each balloon can be thrown before it bursts... all over the child on the receiving end!

TRAIL ABOUT TOWN

DIFFICULTY: ||||

Write clues and riddles about the local area, culminating in a mystery destination, such as a café or ice cream parlour. Two teams could battle it out to get to the final meeting point, and you could draft in local shopkeepers or neighbours who you know well to have clues hidden in their shop or front gardens.

What you'll need

- The imagination to come up with the clues
- An accompanying adult for each team if participants aren't old enough to be out alone

---

This approach can also work well to liven up sightseeing on holidays or days out.

GO ON A NIGHT HIKE

DIFFICULTY: ▮▮▯▯▯

A forest or woodland comes alive in a different way after sunset – creep around by torchlight and see if there are nocturnal creatures about, look at how very different things seem by moonlight, marvel at the starry sky (see page 105). Some nature reserves and city parks organize family hikes after dark – bat and historical walks are popular. Better for older children – little ones might become too weary to walk after their usual bedtime.

What you'll need

- Torches
- A suitable location
- The opportunity to sleep later, if possible, the next day to fend off tiredness

---

Whatever the season and weather, there are different sights and sounds to be seen and heard after dark compared to day.

WILD SWIMMING

DIFFICULTY: ıııı|

Mix it up by getting proficient swimmers to skip the local pool for a river, lake or the sea on a warm day – there are lots of safe, clean places dotted about the country. Definitely not one for children fresh out of armbands, but a carefully chosen spot with copious adult supervision shouldn't be hazardous.

What you'll need

- Towels, a flask with a warm drink and warmer clothes than the weather suggests to get body temperatures up afterwards – even if the air is mild, the water might still be chilly.

Wild swimming allows children to experience often beautiful natural environments – much more inspiring than the usual busy, chlorine-filled swimming pool.

TEPEE TIME

DIFFICULTY: ▮▮▮▯▯

Putting up a garden tepee is surprisingly simple. Place six bamboo canes/stakes in a semi-circle about 60 cm apart, and push each around 2 cm into the ground. Gently draw the tops together, then tie with string so you have a tepee-shaped frame. Fix your sheet in place with clothes pegs, and job done. Adding a blanket as a ground sheet and some cushions will give a "glamping" feel.

What you'll need

- String
- 6 x 5-ft or 6-ft bamboo canes (from a garden centre if you haven't got any)
- An old double sheet
- Clothes pegs
- A blanket and some cushions

GO FOR A LEFT/RIGHT WALK

DIFFICULTY: ●○○○○

From your front door take it in turns to say left or right so that each time you approach a left-hand or right-hand turn, you take the suggested direction... you'll go on a walk that you've possibly never been on before.

What you'll need

- Yourselves!

Such a simple idea – not to mention slightly silly – but there's something indulgent in going on a completely pointless walk in the context of our busy modern lives.

GEOCACHING

DIFFICULTY: ▮▮▮▯▯

This modern take on a treasure hunt is a popular way to liven up hiking. You search for a "cache" hidden by others and when you find it, sign the logbook, take an item and replace the cache with one of your own. There are lots of caches around and each has information online, often with details of whether it's child-friendly and the difficulty of finding it. Although geocaching requires the use of a gadget, it helps the user get out in the real world. It's a wonderful family activity but is equally something older teens can do as a group on their own.

What you'll need

- A geocache app and GPS facility on a smartphone, or a handheld GPS device
- A "cache" item, such as a small pack of cards or toy, to replace the one you take (or you can just leave it behind)

EVENING STORYTELLING AROUND A CAMPFIRE

DIFFICULTY: ▋▋▋▁▁

You don't need to be out in the wilderness camping, or camping at all, for this – a safe and suitable place to build a campfire will do (or use a low, fire-pit style barbecue in the garden). Toast marshmallows and make up silly or spooky stories as a group – one person starts things off and everyone else adds a line at a time in turn. See where the story takes you...

What you'll need

- Marshmallows
- Skewers to put them onto
- Wood and a lighter/matches for a campfire or barbecue
- An adult to supervise

WATER SLIDING

DIFFICULTY:
(IF SHOP-BOUGHT) ▮▮▯▯▯ **(IF DIY)** ▮▮▮▮▮

You can buy water slides from toy shops or make one: take a roll of heavy duty bin bags or a plastic tarpaulin, lay them/it on the grass, ideally down a slope, and leave the hosepipe running onto it (provided there isn't a water shortage). You might need to weigh down the corners – choose something that won't hurt sliders in a collision. Works well with an inflatable boogie board/small airbed for the sliding.

What you'll need

- A shop-bought water slide kit
- A small inflatable airbed/board to slide on

For DIYers:

- A hosepipe
- A roll of plastic or bin liners
- A small inflatable airbed/board to slide on

BACK GARDEN BOWLING "ALLEY"

DIFFICULTY: ●●○○○

Who needs expensive bowling alleys when you can put together your own for free (and as a bonus you don't need to wear those funny shoes)? Raid the recycling bin (ask the neighbours if you can pilfer from theirs too) and fill ten or 12 used plastic bottles with water and an optional few drops of different shades of food colouring for a colour-coded points scheme. Place the bottles in the usual triangular formation on a flat strip of ground, grab the ball and await those first shouts of "Strike!"

What you'll need

- Plastic bottles
- A mid-sized ball
- Food colouring (optional)
- Mark standing spots for different age players with a couple of rulers or some tape

GO CRABBING

DIFFICULTY: ▍▍▍▎▎

Kids getting crabby indoors? Head for the seaside and see what they can catch – even if it's nothing much, they'll enjoy trying and scoffing the essential "ice cream on a seaside day out" afterwards. We're told by folk in the know that crabs like to hang out around rock pools, harbour walls and piers – pick your destination with that in mind.

What you'll need

- Some string
- A stone to weigh the string down
- Bait (crabs like bits of chicken, fish or raw bacon)
- A bucket of water to put the crabs in until they're set free again

---

Don't leave crabs in a bucket for too long – return them to the water as soon as possible.

DAISY CHAIN DECORATIONS

DIFFICULTY: ❚❚◳◳◳

Extremely unlikely to drag the average *Call of Duty* player from their screen, but for gentler souls who appreciate pretty things, making daisy chains is a charming way to create bracelets and garlands and triggers a nostalgia trip for many of us parents.

What you'll need

- Daisies galore
- A thumbnail to pierce stems

If this brings back childhood memories, use it as a cue to talk about what else you used to get up to – younger ones will love hearing about "the olden days" (even if it wasn't that long ago to us, it's practically ancient history to them).

Get Outdoors

FLY A KITE SOMEWHERE BRIGHT, BREEZY AND BEAUTIFUL

DIFFICULTY: ▮▮▯▯▯

Find an exposed hill or a breezy beach, run along and let your kite soar! If you don't own a kite, it's possible to knock one up out of sticks or straws, plastic bags and string, although don't bank on it lasting the duration. If you can find a kite-flying event to join in with, even better – they can be quite a spectacle.

What you'll need

- A kite
- A breezy day (wind speeds of 5 to 25 mph are optimal)
- A nice open space – the park, a field, or the beach – without any overhead wires for the kite to collide with

---

It's said that if you build a love of nature in your children before the age of 12, you'll create a lifelong passion for the outdoors.

CLOUD SPOTTING

DIFFICULTY: ●○○○○

Lying down on the grass watching clouds sail by can be both mesmerizing and relaxing. What can they spot in the shapes? Does that one over there look like a face or the one beside it resemble a cat? Talk about different cloud formations, too, and the weather they're associated with – knowing their stratus from their cumulonimbus helps kids get savvy about weather conditions.

What you'll need

- A cloudy but not fully overcast day
- A guide to cloud formations if you don't know them yourself
- A waterproof blanket if the ground's damp

If they go quiet, leave them to relax and contemplate – that's what this "activity" is about: a bit of inactivity.

Get Outdoors

GO PUDDLE JUMPING AND GET THOROUGHLY WET AND MUDDY

DIFFICULTY: ●○○○○

A bit of rain never hurt anyone, and the mud, well, it'll wash off! And in the process of getting utterly soaked and mucky, they'll have a ball; it's liberating not to have parents yelling "don't get too dirty" for a change and positively encouraging the grubbiness fest.

What you'll need

- A muddy, wet day
- Wellies
- Waterproofs

No such thing as bad weather,
only inappropriate clothes!

ROUNDERS IN THE PARK

DIFFICULTY: ◼◼◻◻◻

Enduringly popular with sporty and rather less sporty types, this classic bat and ball game is a sociable way to get everyone running about. It can be enjoyed by players of mixed ages (as long as they're old enough to whack a ball or catch) and skills but you do need a small crowd, so this is best for when you're meeting up with other families or for a larger group of kids.

What you'll need

- A rounders bat and ball
- A few sweaters/bean bags for the bases
- At least 12 people in total to make for a decent game

If your children prefer something a little more sedate, boules is a great alternative that can be played in the garden or park.

VISIT A PICK-YOUR-OWN FARM

DIFFICULTY: ●●○○○

Fresh air and a reminder that food doesn't magically appear on supermarket shelves all packaged up. Pick-your-own fruit and veg farms are at their best in summer and early autumn – most provide information on what's available for harvesting at any one time. PYO farms offer seasonal produce that is as fresh as you can get, with low food-to-plate miles.

What you'll need

- Some money to pay for produce picked – most farms provide bags or containers

---

Suggest older offspring research dishes they can cook up with the fruits or veg of their labour from the PYO farm.

CONKER CHAMPIONSHIPS

DIFFICULTY: ▮▮▯▯▯

This is a timeless autumn activity: hunt for the biggest, shiniest conkers and then hold a belting conker fight. Conker aficionados maximize their chances of victory by picking large, symmetrical and uncracked conkers and hardening them in the oven for a short while, soaking them in vinegar or freezing them overnight and rolling them in hand cream (yes, really). Then let battle commence!

What you'll need

- Conkers
- Strong string (about 25 cm for each)
- Something to pierce a hole through the conker to thread the string through – it might be preferable to have an adult to do this for them

AMAZING MAZES

DIFFICULTY: ❙❙❘❘❘

There are mazes made of maize crops or traditional versions created with hedges and bushes up and down the country. If there are enough of you, work in teams of two or more (younger kids might need to be accompanied by an adult) and compete to see who can get out first.

What you'll need

- A maze. Traditional mazes can be found at some historical properties and maize versions at some farms seasonally.

If your child enjoyed exploring a real maze, introduce them to paper versions back home – downloadable online and great for working their brains.

WATER PISTOL SHOOTING RANGE

DIFFICULTY: ▮▮▯▯▯

Stick a row of golf tees firmly onto a flat surface with Blu-tack or push them into the top of a cardboard box – they must be vertical. Then balance a ping-pong ball upon each tee. Players need to knock the balls off the tees with water from a water pistol to score points. Upscale this if the children have got hefty water guns and use bigger or heavier targets (plastic bottles with water in or a row of rubber ducks or larger balls) or put them further away.

What you'll need

- One or two small water pistols, ping-pong balls, golf tees, Blu-tack, a cardboard box, plus a flat surface, e.g. a garden table

---

Great for dexterity and refreshing on a hot day.

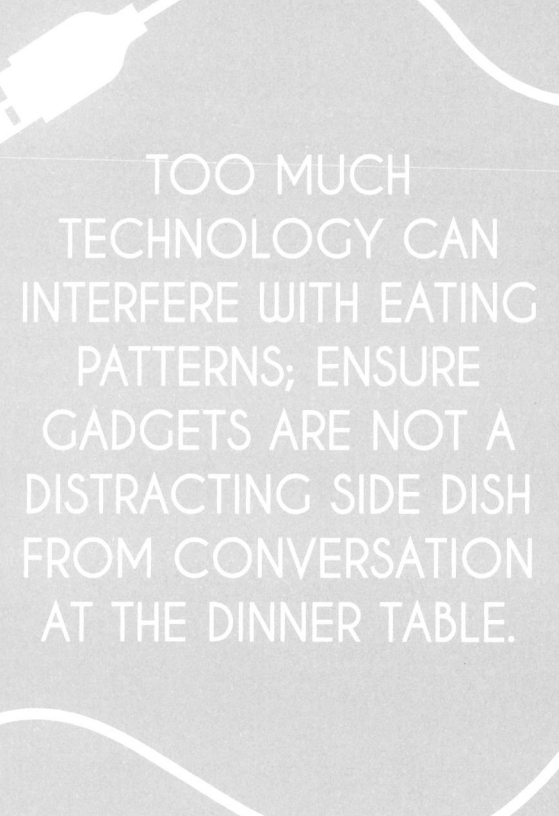

TOO MUCH TECHNOLOGY CAN INTERFERE WITH EATING PATTERNS; ENSURE GADGETS ARE NOT A DISTRACTING SIDE DISH FROM CONVERSATION AT THE DINNER TABLE.

ARTY AND CRAFTY

TABLET

GLITTER

Arty and Crafty

CARDBOARD BOX CRAFTING

DIFFICULTY: ▋▋▏▏▏

It's a box, a box made of cardboard – could it get any duller? But that box might just have new life awaiting it as something else, anything else, whatever a child's imagination comes up with. Hand them a sturdy box, plus a pile of props, and see what they create – a bed, a cupboard, a shop, a theatre, an oven, a car, a teddy bear hospital...

What you'll need

- A box – the bigger the better
- Masking or parcel tape
- Large marker pens for decoration
- A cutting tool (for use by an adult depending on their age) for windows, doors, etc.

The simplest things can breed imagination and creativity – leave children to make their own minds up about what their box will be.

CREATE A SLOGAN T-SHIRT

DIFFICULTY:

Plain T-shirts can be picked up for a small price, so why not have them make one their own by adding a quote from a speech, book or poem. Something funny, beautiful or inspiring which others will take note of. They'll need to research, think through and hopefully discuss exactly what is worthy of their T-shirt. Other ideas for decoration include sewing or sticking on braids, ribbons, etc. or using fabric paint and stencils.

What you'll need

- A plain white or pale T-shirt
- A fabric or laundry pen and items for decorating
- Books, films or (dare we say it) internet gadgets for research

---

Encourage discussion of which quote or poem is best and why.

GET CROCHETING

DIFFICULTY: ▮▮▮▮▯

If they bought into the loom band craze in recent years, then crocheting is a natural next step. OK, it's probably not going to excite a completely un-crafty kid, but the satisfaction of learning to turn a ball of yarn into a scarf or even a funky cover for their beloved gadgets is considerable. They might get hooked…

What you'll need

- Yarn
- Crochet hook
- A pattern or two (or buy a crochet kit for kids) – you could look for tutorials online just to start them off

---

Crochet: definitely not just for grannies!

RUBBER STAMP LETTERS

DIFFICULTY: ▮▮▯▯▯

There's something charmingly old-school about a message made with stamp letters. Friends could write notes to each other and then post them to their respective homes. Come December, get some festive picture stamps, too, and they can create Christmas cards with a personal touch.

What you'll need

- A stamp and ink pad set from a craft or toy shop
- Some coloured paper or blank greeting cards
- Envelopes

The more the world flings itself into digital messaging, the more retro and exciting receiving a proper letter or postcard seems.

Arty and Crafty

CUSTOMIZE CANVAS PLIMSOLLS

DIFFICULTY: ■■■□□

Fashion forward crafty kids will love designing a pair of unique couture plimsolls – literally a blank canvas to let their creative juices run wild with. They might not prove waterproof but for dry days they'll be the coolest shoes in town.

What you'll need

- A pair of canvas plimsolls (clothing discount retailers sell them cheaply)
- PVA glue
- Acrylic paint
- A wide brush
- Fabric pens
- Stick-on beads and serious amounts of glitter (optional)
- Masking tape for neatening edges of different sections or stripes

PAPER MARBLING

DIFFICULTY: ●●○○○

This centuries-old art produces beautiful results. Pour water 1 cm to 2 cm deep into a tray, add blobs of marbling ink, then swirl away with a stick/pencil. Lay paper flat on (not under) the water, before carefully lifting and then drying it face up on newspaper. Gorgeous for notebook coverings or wrapping paper.

What you'll need

- A large tray with deep sides – an old roasting tin or disposable tray
- Marbling paint/ink
- Water
- Card or thick paper that fits in the tray
- A pencil, stick or comb to create swirls

Creating the marble swirls and patterns can be strangely relaxing and quite hypnotic.

Arty and Crafty

LIFE-SIZE SELF-PORTRAITS

DIFFICULTY:

One person lies down on a large sheet of paper, while another draws their outline. Once that's done they can then draw on their own details, self-portrait-style – eyes, mouth, clothing – before colouring in/painting.

What you'll need

- A roll of wallpaper liner paper or similar large, thick paper (too thin and it might tear)
- Paints/colouring pens and washable markers for the outline

You could turn the self-portraits into cardboard cut-outs – sticking the paper to sturdy card and cutting around the edge of the outline with heavy duty scissors.

HOME-MADE SNOW DOUGH

DIFFICULTY: ▮▯▯▯▯

Mix up snow dough (softer than play dough but still mouldable) with them before letting little ones loose to create wintry scenes or simply enjoy playing with its lovely squishy texture. Add food colouring for brightness or glitter for sparkles and provide a few tools for making shapes and patterns. Use 8 cups of plain flour, add 1 cup of baby oil and stir. Watch out: this can get messy!

What you'll need

- A large tub or bowl
- Flour
- Baby oil (or vegetable oil, if toddlers try to eat the dough)
- Food colouring or glitter (optional)
- Tools

Softer and squashier than play dough, small hands can mould, sculpt and smooth it away.

OUTDOOR FLOOR CHALKING

DIFFICULTY: ●○○○○

There's a cheeky freedom to drawing on floors, even if they're outside on the terrace, patio or driveway (just make sure smaller children know the difference between this versus marker pens on the carpet). No hard surfaces in the garden? Chalk on pavements instead – if neighbours get grumpy, reassure them it'll wash away when it rains (or sneak out later with a watering can – for the chalk, not to pour over grouchy neighbours!).

What you'll need

- Various colours of chalk
- A hard outdoor surface

Create a chalk hopscotch grid, too, and they can hop and skip along – they'll need a marker (coin, stone or bean bag) for this.

DRAW A FUNKY HAND

DIFFICULTY: ▮▮▯▯▯

Draw around the outline of your hand, then create mehndi-style henna designs or funky intricate doodles and patterns in it, or try to make it look three-dimensional with curves and lines. A simple, although less time-consuming, idea is to colour the hand in with one bright and bold colour and the surrounding paper with a contrasting one.

For a family memento or gift for grandparents, add several members of the family's hand outlines to one larger piece of paper and get each person to colour in and decorate their own hand.

What you'll need

- A4 paper
- Colouring pens
- Pencils

Arty and Crafty

PAPER PEOPLE CHAINS

DIFFICULTY: ∎∎∎☐☐

Another old-fashioned activity that retains allure for craftier kids. Take a longish strip of paper (or cut an A4 page in half lengthways), fold the sheet up, concertina-style, then draw half a person-shaped outline at the folded side. Cut around the outline but not at the folded side, unfold, and voilà – a cute paper doll chain ready to decorate.

What you'll need

- Paper
- Pencil
- Colouring pens/paint for decoration
- Scissors that are tough enough to cut through a few layers of paper (for younger children, it might be best for you to do this bit)

MAKE A MINI PARACHUTE

DIFFICULTY: ▮▮▯▯▯

You can buy these but it's satisfying and not difficult to make your own. Cut a plastic bag into a rectangle or square, add small holes to each corner, take four equal lengths of string and feed one through each hole in the bag and then stick each piece to a different corner of an empty yoghurt pot. Put an uncooked egg in the pot to see if it can fall from window to ground unbroken!

What you'll need

- A plastic bag
- Clean, empty yoghurt pot
- String or wool
- Sticky tape
- Scissors
- Cargo or robust plastic figurines as passengers (optional)
- A window

PRESS FLOWERS AND LEAVES

DIFFICULTY: ❚❚❘❘❘

Take a selection of freshly picked flowers (flatter is better than chunky) and leaves, dry them with a cloth or tissue, pop them between the pages of a book lined with some thick paper, close the book and then weigh it down with something heavy. Wait two to four weeks – a long time – and then you'll be ready to make some pictures. A charming, traditional activity, but not for the impatient!

What you'll need

- A book
- A heavy weight
- Some nice thick paper (blotting, cartridge or watercolour is best)
- A selection of pretty flowers and leaves

UPCYCLE OLD CLOTHES

DIFFICULTY:
(BASIC) ▮▮▮▯▯   (ADVANCED) ▮▮▮▮▮

Aspiring designers can grab garments from local charity shops or the back of the wardrobe and customize them with their own unique brand of chic. Add lace, studs or glitter to denim, chop off sleeves or trouser legs or change necklines.

What you'll need

- Cheap or second-hand clothing
- Ribbon
- Lace
- Buttons
- Fabric paint
- Pens
- Dye
- Scissors
- A sewing kit

Arty and Crafty

HANDMADE GREETINGS CARDS

DIFFICULTY:
(BASIC) ιι❘❘❘ (ADVANCED) ιιιιι

Relatives will surely appreciate the efforts that go into handmade cards, which can be personalized to the recipient too. Entrepreneurial offspring could sell their card creations at school fairs or elsewhere.

What you'll need

- Blank cards and envelopes from stationery or art/craft shops (the thicker the card the better)
- Glue
- Glitter
- Metallic pens
- Festive and alphabet stamp and ink pads
- Scraps of wrapping and tissue paper, wallpaper or coloured card

ORGANIZE SOME ORIGAMI

DIFFICULTY: ▮▮▮▯▯

Basic origami tutorials abound in books and online. Little hats, boats, stars and animals can be knocked up with just a few folds when you know how. A traditional favourite grown-ups might recall is the fortune teller, with four quarters you move with your fingers, each numbered and corresponding to statements about the future underneath, e.g. "you will be rich" or "your parents will allow you unlimited screen time forever…"

What you'll need

- Paper
- Origami instructions – either a book or printed from the internet by parents

---

Works well for travelling as all you need is some paper and a small flat surface to work on.

Arty and Crafty

MAKE A MARBLE RUN

DIFFICULTY: ❙❙❙❘❘

Again, you can buy these in the shops and they're very engaging in themselves but making your own is even more so. You're looking to create a series of ramps with smooth runs for the marbles to tumble down, plus holes for them to fall through onto further ramps below. Taking the run down a staircase adds extra fun to this.

What you'll need

- A pile of plastic and cardboard boxes
- Kitchen or toilet paper tubes
- Heavyweight tape, e.g. duct tape, scissors
- Some marbles

If you've got enough people around to make it work, two teams could compete to create the longest working run – time how long the marble goes without stopping from start to finish.

NEWSPAPER FASHION SHOW

DIFFICULTY: ▮▮▮▮▯

Good for a gaggle of pre-teens or teens working in pairs; one person stands whilst the other "dresses" them using newspaper, tape and scissors alone, then swap over if desired. Create a catwalk in the living room and stage a fashion show with music at the end to show off their creations.

What you'll need

- Tons of newspapers
- Scissors
- Masking tape
- Paint to add colour (optional)

A photographer or two from among the group could take snaps as the "models" strut their stuff before the optional "after show party".

Arty and Crafty

TIE-DYE T-SHIRTS

DIFFICULTY: ●●●○○

Come over all "groovy, baby" with a Seventies-style tie-dye shirt. They're easy to create with the basic technique of tying on string or using rubber bands to make dye-free rings in the fabric. As well as T-shirts, tea towels, pairs of jeans or old pillowcases can be jazzed up – almost anything goes.

What you'll need

- Plain white T-shirts or other items (100 per cent cotton takes on colours the best)
- Fabric dye
- A bucket or washing up bowl (be aware that it might get stained)
- Rubber bands or string
- Rubber gloves
- Some dyes also require salt – check the packaging

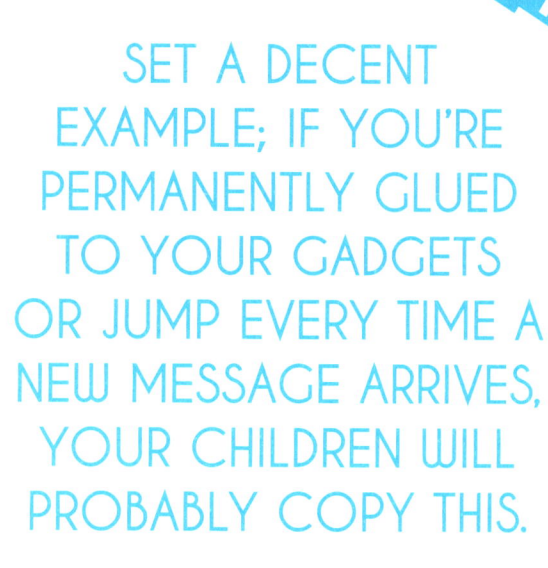

SET A DECENT EXAMPLE; IF YOU'RE PERMANENTLY GLUED TO YOUR GADGETS OR JUMP EVERY TIME A NEW MESSAGE ARRIVES, YOUR CHILDREN WILL PROBABLY COPY THIS.

FOOD AND COOKING

THE GREAT FAMILY BAKE OFF (AND CAKE SCOFF AFTERWARDS)

DIFFICULTY:
(BAKING) ▮▮▮▯▯   (SCOFFING) ▯▯▯▯▯

Hold a home version of *Bake Off* with friends or relatives and a retro tea party session afterwards to judge who does the best biscuits or the finest fondant fancies. Think pink lemonade, floral napkins, proper teapots and fancy cake stands to showcase their creations.

What you'll need

- Baking ingredients
- Recipes
- Kitchen gear

Keen older cooks could take charge of birthday cake making and decorating – a home-made cake will invariably delight recipients.

Food and Cooking

GET JAMMING

DIFFICULTY: ▮▮▮▮▯

More of a joint activity as the jam can get dangerously hot, but this is brilliant for dealing with fruit overload after foraging or visiting a pick-your-own farm (see pages 63 and 94). Experiment with different combinations and more unusual flavours, such as melon or rhubarb.

What you'll need

- Piles of fruit
- Preserving sugar
- A large sturdy saucepan or preserving pan
- Sterilized jam jars with lids
- A jam-making thermometer

Home-made jams packaged up prettily make a lovely gift – make your own labels with brown paper luggage labels and string for a pared down look.

MAKE YOUR OWN PIZZA

DIFFICULTY: ▮▮▯▯▯

The almost universal popularity of pizza means it's a sneaky way to tempt reluctant cooks into the kitchen. As well as doing all the kneading and rolling of dough, get them to think up new topping combinations and schedule some pizza-themed games for during the dough proving phase.

What you'll need

- Dough
- Topping ingredients
- Rolling pin
- Baking tray

Take this one step further by decorating the kitchen/dining area as a pizzeria, with menus and home-made Italian flags.

Food and Cooking

COME DINE WITH US

DIFFICULTY: ιιιll

Split into teams – these could each have a parent and a child or be from a gang of teenage friends – and stage a cooking competition. Each Friday or Saturday evening, one team makes dinner and the others get to judge their culinary prowess and hosting skills. If you all enjoy it the first time, introduce themes for future rounds. The competition will be heating up as well as the nosh...

What you'll need

- Ingredients
- Recipes
- Kitchens

This one really gets everyone chatting – but remember: no screens at the table. One idea to get people talking is to blindfold the diners at the table before food is served and then get them to guess what it is.

GO FORAGING...

DIFFICULTY: ▮▮▯▯▯

From blackberries and elderberries to sloes and rosehips, at the right time of year a bit of foraging can uncover all manner of edible goodies, and the kids will enjoy spotting the best locations and comparing hauls.

Of course, only pick and eat something if you are 100 per cent sure you've identified it correctly and try not to strip plants bare so local wildlife gets its share too.

What you'll need

- A suitable location – this needn't be deepest countryside: for example, blackberries can often be found in urban green spaces too
- Bags/baskets
- Long trousers in case you're picking among prickly bushes

Food and Cooking

... THEN MAKE THREE DIFFERENT THINGS WITH YOUR FINDS

DIFFICULTY:

You've foraged the food, now challenge them to research and make three things with each ingredient. So, for blackberries, how about a pie, smoothie and fruit fool? Rosehips could be turned into jam, syrup and even a skincare oil. Apples can be made into juice, crumble and a tart.

What you'll need

- Recipes
- A pile of foraged goods
- Other necessary ingredients

As a bonus, this gets them consuming more of their five a day – result!

MAKE ICE CREAM

DIFFICULTY: ▮▮▮▯▯

An activity to delight all ages – who doesn't love ice cream? Once the base recipe has been mastered, experiment with new flavours and textures, or move on to sorbets.

Don't forget the toppings: sprinkles, mini-marshmallows and chocolate flakes!

What you'll need

- A freezer or ice cream making machine
- Relevant ingredients
- Some ice cream parlour-style bowls
- Spoons for serving

For a shortcut and instant gelato gratification, look up an "ice cream in a bag" recipe – a super-quick method using ice cubes and zipper storage bags.

Food and Cooking

BECOME SUSHI CHEFS

DIFFICULTY: ▍▍▍▎▁

One for the more sophisticated palate but all the rolling, dipping, wrapping and chopping (for those old enough to handle knives safely) is supremely satisfying and the finished product looks fabulously impressive. And it's healthy too!

What you'll need

- Typical ingredients include nori sheets, sushi rice, rice wine vinegar and light soy sauce
- For protein and veg elements, smoked salmon, cucumber, avocado, crab meat and tuna are popular

---

Visiting a Japanese food shop can be interesting but if there isn't one nearby, most large supermarkets should have the necessary ingredients for basic sushi recipes.

BLINDFOLD FEAST

DIFFICULTY: ●●○○○

Set up a feast from unusual foods in the fridge or cupboards, blindfold friends or family and get them to identify the items by taste. Make sure it's all edible and not too revolting; leaving out the *I'm a Celebrity*-style live locusts could be wise.

What you'll need

- Assorted foodstuffs – both familiar and more mysterious
- A tray
- Some small pots to put each item into

A wacky way to encourage fussy eaters to try new foods – they won't like them all but at least they'll have given them a go.

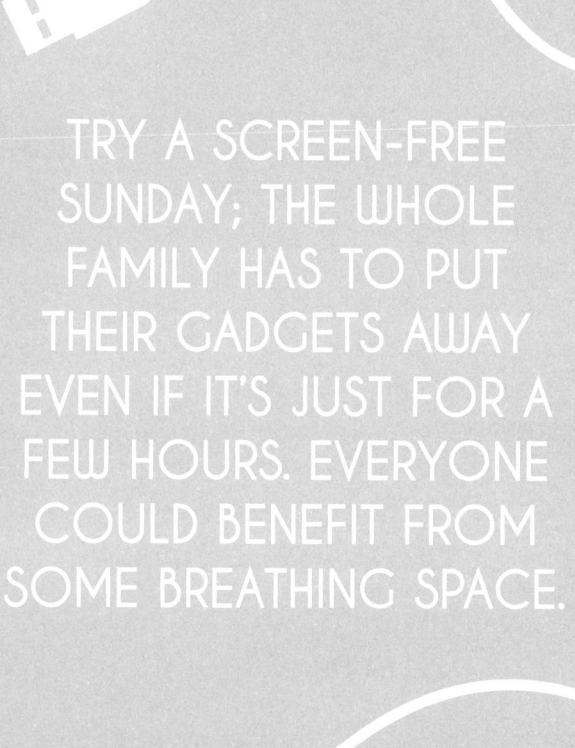

SCIENCE AND NATURE

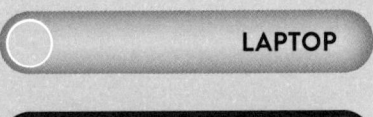

Science and Nature

GROW A GROSS MOULD GARDEN

DIFFICULTY: ●○○○○

Revolting and fascinating in equal measure: your kids will see how the furry white and green stuff develops and which foods get grossest quickest. Put different food scraps in clean jars that you won't want to reuse afterwards (you MUST throw them away/put them in the recycling at the end and do not open them once the mould has arrived), and see how the mould grows, checking daily over a couple of weeks.

What you'll need

- Several clean jars
- Tape to seal the jars
- Sticky labels to mark the jars as "mould gardens – DO NOT OPEN... EVER"
- Chunks of several foods (e.g. orange peel, bread, but not meat or fish as these will get too stinky)

Kids could take daily photos to document the mould's growth.

BECOME WEATHER REPORTERS

DIFFICULTY: ▮▮▯▯▯

Create a home weather station and monitor the change in seasons in a diary. As well as making a rain gauge and using a thermometer, junior weather reporters might look up the Beaufort scale to assess winds (they could draw a chart with examples if they're arty). It will entice them outdoors to check conditions every day, come rain or shine.

What you'll need

- A large empty drinks bottle for the rain gauge
- A ruler
- Tape
- Scissors
- A pencil
- A thermometer
- Information on the Beaufort scale
- A diary/notepad

Science and Nature

COLA BOTTLE SCIENCE

DIFFICULTY: ●○○○○

A simple experiment that's a real blast. Grab a bottle of cola (diet will be less sticky to clear up post-eruption) and some Mentos sweets. You can use just one Mentos but the more the merrier; pop several into a small tube and let them fall into the bottle at the same time to maximize the effect. Absolutely best done outdoors for obvious reasons and make sure you run away quickly once the sweets go in.

What you'll need

- A bottle of cola
- A packet of Mentos
- Fizzy drinks of different kinds and different sweets could be tried to expand the experiment – which will create the tallest plume?

Afterwards, send curious kids off to research the science behind the explosive reaction.

CREEPY-CRAWLY CATCHER

DIFFICULTY: ▮▮▯▯▯

Many a small child is enthralled by bugs and ants; this quick-to-make creepy-crawly catcher creates a temporary habitat for your child to observe them in.

Take a clean, empty plastic berry container, remove any label, then craft a door in the lid by cutting around three sides, so it can be lifted up and down. Tape around all the edges of the box lid, and job done... time to get out hunting for those bugs, although don't forget to set them free at the end (outside!).

What you'll need

- A berry container
- Masking tape
- Scissors and a grown-up to do the cutting of the door (tape over any sharp edges on the cut plastic too)

Science and Nature

STARRY, STARRY NIGHTS

DIFFICULTY: ■□□□□

Research the main constellations and roll out some facts to add interest, e.g. how when we gaze at the stars, we're looking into the past: the stars are so far away, their light has only just reached Earth and some might not even exist by now. If the sky's particularly clear and you're away from light pollution, shooting stars can be especially thrilling for kids to see.

What you'll need

- A clear evening in a place with little or no light pollution
- Information on constellations if you aren't familiar with them

---

There's something awe-inspiring about gazing up at a starry sky.

GARDEN (OR PARK) SCAVENGER HUNT

DIFFICULTY: ■■□□□

Using a piece of chalk on a terrace or paved area in your garden, write a selection of items you want the children to find. Or grab a pen and paper and write a list for the park. Specify anything and everything: feathers, pine cones, rose petals, daisies, stones or leaves of a particular shape, clover. Get them to be mindful of what's around them as they search for their treasure.

What you'll need

- A container to stow the evidence in if at the park
- At home you could create a circle on the terrace/paving for each item to be placed into

---

This activity has them learning about plants and nature and running round in the fresh air all at the same time.

Science and Nature

FOREVER BLOWING (GIANT) BUBBLES

DIFFICULTY: ●●●○○

Most kids have had fun bubble blowing on a small scale, but supersize the bubbles and you supersize the laughs. To make the bubble mix, stir the ingredients together, then, if possible, leave it overnight in a large tray/bowl. To make your bubble wand, shape an old wire coat hanger into a circle (as best you can) and cover the hook's sharp end with masking tape so no one loses an eye. Choose a still day as wind will scupper efforts.

What you'll need

For the bubble mix:
- 1 litre of water, 70 ml of washing up liquid, 25 ml glycerine (sold in chemists or supermarkets), a large tray/bowl

For the bubble wand:
- An old wire coat hanger
- Masking tape

STICK AND MARSHMALLOW TOWER BUILDING

DIFFICULTY: ▮▮▯▯▯

Get them honing their construction skills and pondering physics: see how tall a tower they can build using toothpicks or spaghetti stuck together with marshmallows, fashioned into piles of pyramids. It's a sticky, tricky task, not least because you've got to ensure the construction workers don't scoff half the building materials.

What you'll need

- A lot of marshmallows
- Dry spaghetti or several packs of toothpicks

Turn this into a competition with teams battling to build the tallest tower and test robustness by making them place an egg at the top.

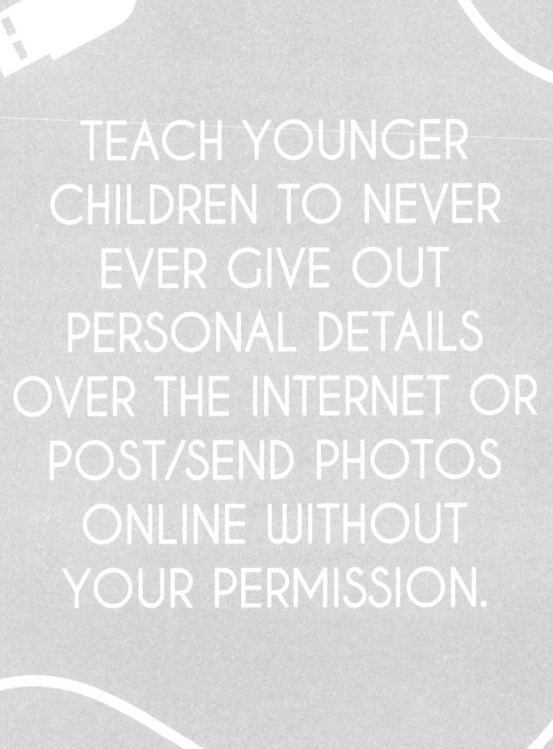

ACTIVITIES ON THE GO

SPOTIFY

SPONTANEITY

THE MEMORY GAME

DIFFICULTY: ●○○○○

You probably remember this old chestnut (if you don't, your memory might not be up to playing...): one person starts off saying "I went to the shops and bought" and adds the name of something, and then each of the other players has to add an item in turn and recall all the previous ones too. First to mess up and forget is out.

What you'll need

- A half-decent memory
- At least two people

Variations on this include "I went on holiday and I packed...", "I went to school and did..." and "I met a footballer/celebrity called...", depending on age and interests.

PENCIL AND PAPER GAMES

DIFFICULTY: ▮▮▯▯▯

Dots and boxes, battleships, hangman, noughts and crosses: all still appealing ways to stay occupied offline. Invest a little time explaining the rules, and bingo (well, actually not bingo), you've got a load of sociable games your kids can do anywhere, with nothing more than a pen/pencil and the back of an envelope or a paper napkin.

What you'll need

- Pencil or pen
- Some paper

They might lack the whizzy, super-fast action and fancy graphics of gaming, but these are wholesome and can truly be played anywhere, especially if you've forgotten the tablet or don't want to hand over your smartphone.

20 QUESTIONS/ANIMAL, VEGETABLE OR MINERAL

DIFFICULTY: ●○○○○

One player, the "chooser", thinks of an object and can only let the other player(s) know if it's an animal, vegetable or mineral in nature. Guessers then have 20 questions that the chooser can only respond to with a "yes" or "no". If they haven't got to the answer within those 20 questions, the chooser wins.

What you'll need

- Nothing!

Sometimes suggestions such as this will be met with unenthusiastic groans, but once they give it a go, even the most plugged-in kids might surprise themselves and find that non-digital games can be OK too.

WOULD YOU RATHER...

DIFFICULTY: ●○○○○

Each person takes it in turns to ask the others which of two bad, mad or fantastic options they'd prefer. It could be as simple as "Would you rather marry Harry Styles or Timothée Chalamet?" or as weird as "Would you rather be invisible or be able to fly?"

Be warned: this one can get seriously silly!

What you'll need

- Nothing!

A fantastic conversation starter that can provide insights into your child's thinking.

DESERT ISLAND DISCS

DIFFICULTY: ●○○○○

Assuming your kids don't listen to the famous BBC Radio 4 programme and might not even get the reference to discs meaning music, this might require some explaining. So, you're a shipwrecked castaway and must name eight pieces of music, one book and a luxury item that will help ease life on that desert island. Adapt it if your kids aren't into music – they could name toys, food or friends to take.

What you'll need

- Again, nothing!

Pad things out by making players create fantastical stories about how they ended up on the island and how they might escape as well. They could perhaps pick three items to enable that escape and then describe how they'd do it.

BEATBOX BAND

DIFFICULTY: ▮▮▮▯▯

If you aren't down with the kids on this, beatbox is a kind of modern, hip-hop take on a cappella. A group works together to make music just with their voices and bodies, but there are no rules here, so add in a bit of table or tin lid drumming, finger clicking and clapping and see what tunes come out.

What you'll need
- A small group of people
- Some beatbox inspiration from YouTube to get them into the idea

---

A real teamwork task that can be done pretty much anywhere where it won't annoy others around you.

30-DAY PHOTO CHALLENGE

DIFFICULTY: ▮▮▮▯▯

Children must come up with a list of 30 interesting or unusual categories to inspire a photo each day: "my favourite thing", "a view", "words", "the season", "food", "inspired by a song" or "close up", perhaps. The ideas could be more arty and obscure for older children (adjectives and emotions work well here). A little and often project, rather than one that will last hours in one go.

What you'll need

- A camera
- A way of printing the photos at the end to make an album or photobook of the project, as well as potentially posting on social media if they're old enough. A lot of us no longer print photos, so they could also choose their favourite shot of the 30 to frame and put on the wall somewhere.

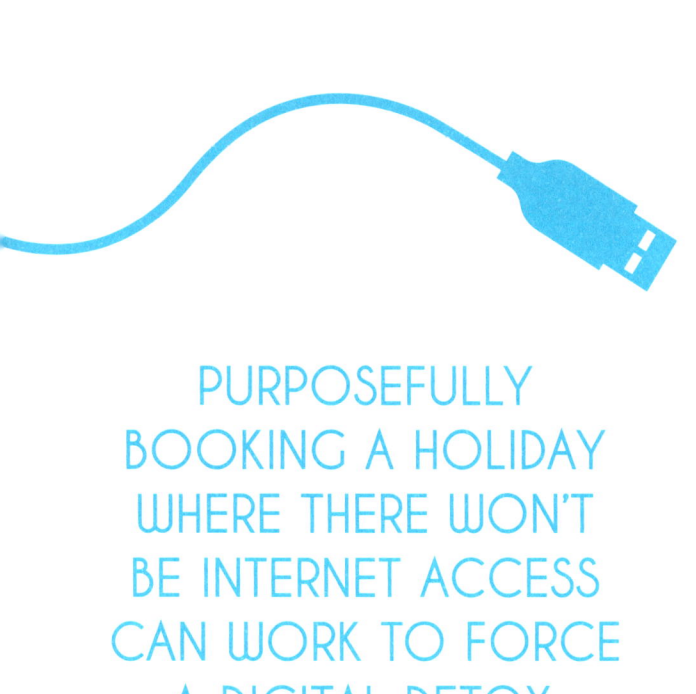

A FEW MORE IDEAS...

- GAMES CONSOLE
- IMAGINATION

PREDICT THEIR OWN FUTURE

DIFFICULTY: ▮▮▯▯▯

Thinking 15 or 20 years on fascinates most children: what will they be doing and what might have changed in daily life with new innovations? Come up with a template together or get them to create one, with categories such as: their job, where they'll live and with whom, their holidays, car and pets. Add the date, and place their predictions in an envelope to keep until they're adults – will they come true?

What you'll need

- Paper
- Pens

For more fun: predict what the wider world will be like sometime in the future – try 20 years ahead. What might change and what could be invented?

A Few More Ideas...

CAR BOOT/GARAGE SALE CLEAR-OUT

DIFFICULTY: ▮▮▯▯▯

Many a modern family is overrun with toys and general kids' stuff. The words "let's have a clear-out" aren't exactly enticing to children, but add in the prospect of flogging all their outgrown and unused gear at a boot sale to create some cash, and they might well come running.

What you'll need

- The fee to pay for a boot sale pitch, or you could do it as a garage/table in the driveway sale and make posters to publicize it

---

Consider encouraging a small donation to charity from the day's takings.

RANDOM ACTS OF KINDNESS DAY

DIFFICULTY: ■■□□□

Your child has to come up with, say, five to ten random kind things to do in a day. How about: delivering homemade biscuits to those lonely elderly neighbours, letting someone else jump a queue, inviting the child who struggles to make friends round, picking litter up? But the activity here is about coming up with the ideas as well as the doing, so let the children think some up themselves.

What you'll need

- A dose of generosity!
- Possibly some money if their acts involve you paying for things or ingredients for baking

---

This is sure to warm their hearts as well as hopefully those of the people on the receiving end.

A Few More Ideas...

START THEIR OWN (VERY SMALL FOR NOW) BUSINESS

DIFFICULTY: ▮▮▯▯▯

Got a budding tycoon in the family? Pocket money-boosters, such as car washing, greetings card making (see page 83) and dog walking (see page 43), are an introduction to the entrepreneurial world and all suitable for teens with a can-do attitude who want to earn some extra cash. If they're making something, eBay and Etsy mean they can sell their wares easily.

What you'll need

- Possibly some leaflets to advertize their goods or services locally (they should make these)
- Raw materials if it involves making something

Ask key business questions – what's different about their product/service, who are their potential customers and how will they advertize to them, can they make a profit?

KEEPING SCREENS IN COMMUNAL AREAS OF THE HOUSE – I.E. NOT IN BEDROOMS – MAKES IT EASIER TO MONITOR WHAT YOUR CHILDREN ARE LOOKING AT AND HOW MUCH THEY'RE ON THEM.

SHUT DOWN: COMPLETE

I hope these activities have given you and your kids a chance to spend time offline with each other and you continue to enjoy spending time away from your screens. Have fun!

Help Your Child Cope with Change

What to Know, Say and Do When Times Are Tough

Liat Hughes Joshi

HELP YOUR CHILD COPE WITH CHANGE

WHAT TO KNOW, SAY AND DO WHEN TIMES ARE TOUGH

Liat Hughes Joshi
Paperback
ISBN: 978-1-80007-194-0

As parents and carers, we try everything in our power to shield our children and prepare them emotionally for disappointments and upsets, but sometimes it can be hard to know what to do for the best. This book offers actionable tips that will give you and your child the tools to navigate these difficult times with kindness and care.

Find out more about the author at
liathughesjoshi.co.uk or follow her @liathughesjoshi

Have you enjoyed this book?

If so, why not write a review on your favourite website?
If you're interested in finding out more about our books,
find us on Facebook at Summersdale Publishers,
on Twitter/X at @Summersdale and on
Instagram and TikTok at @summersdalebooks
and get in touch. We'd love to hear from you!

Thanks very much for buying this Summersdale book.

www.summersdale.com